DIABETIC

RENAL DIET

COOKBOOK

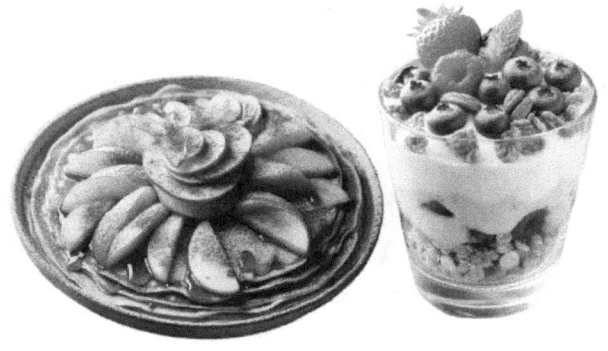

Nutrient-Rich Recipes for Diabetes

Management and Kidney Support

Lanita Cruz

Copyright Page © [2024] Lanita Cruz

TABLE OF CONTENT

Disclaimer

The information provided in this "Diabetic Renal Diet Cookbook" is for educational and informational purposes only. It is not intended as a substitute for professional medical advice, diagnosis, or treatment.

Always seek the advice of your physician or other qualified health provider with any questions you may have regarding a medical condition.

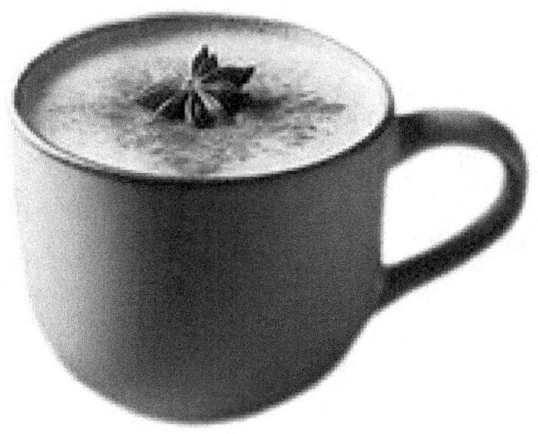

Introduction

If you have Diabetic Renal disease, you may feel overwhelmed by the dietary restrictions you need to follow. You may wonder what you can eat, how much you can eat, and how to prepare your meals.

You may also worry about the long-term effects of your condition on your health and quality of life. But there is hope.

You can take control of your health and manage your condition with a diabetic renal diet.

Welcome to the "Diabetic Renal Diet Cookbook," your essential guide to maintaining a healthy lifestyle while managing both diabetes and renal health.

This cookbook is meticulously crafted to provide you with a collection of delicious recipes tailored to support your well-being.

As diabetes and renal issues often go hand in hand, adopting a thoughtful and balanced approach to your diet is crucial.

In this book, I delved into the principles that form the foundation of the Diabetic Renal Diet, offering valuable insights into the benefits it brings.

Whether you're newly diagnosed or seeking ways to enhance your current dietary habits, embark on this culinary journey with me, discovering not only the foods to enjoy but also those to avoid.

Together, let's navigate the world of flavor and nutrition, empowering you to make informed choices for a more active, healthier, and happier life.

CHAPTER 1

Principles of the Diabetic Renal Diet

1. **Balancing Carbohydrates**: Carbohydrates are the main source of energy for your body, but they also affect your blood sugar levels. You should choose carbohydrates that are low in sugar and high in fiber, such as fruits, vegetables, whole grains, and legumes. You should also limit or avoid carbohydrates that are high in sugar and low in fiber, such as sweets, desserts, sodas, and juices.

2. **Lean Proteins**: Protein is essential for building and repairing your body tissues, but too much protein can strain your kidneys and raise your blood sugar. You should eat moderate amounts of high-quality protein from animal or vegetable sources, such as meat, fish, eggs, milk, beans, lentils, nuts, and seeds.

3. **Incorporating Healthy Fats**: Fats are important for your brain, nerves, and hormones, but some fats are better than others. You should include healthy fats that are rich in omega-3 fatty acids, such as olive

oil, canola oil, flaxseed oil, walnuts, and fatty fish, they provide essential nutrients without contributing to excessive calorie intake, supporting overall well-being. You should also limit or avoid unhealthy fats that are high in saturated fat and cholesterol, such as butter, cream, cheese, bacon, and fatty meats

4. **Mindful Portion Control**: Understanding portion sizes is key to both diabetes and renal health management. This principle aids in weight control, helping you regulate blood sugar levels and reduce stress on the kidneys.

5. **Hydration Importance**: Proper fluid intake is essential for kidney function. Fluids are essential for your body to function properly, but too much fluid can cause swelling, high blood pressure, and heart failure. You should drink enough fluids to keep your urine clear or pale yellow, but not more than your doctor or dietitian recommends.

6. **Sodium Monitoring**: This Diet advocates for a mindful approach to sodium intake, you should avoid or limit foods that are high in sodium. By opting for fresh, whole foods and minimizing

processed options, you can maintain healthy blood pressure levels, crucial for kidney function.

By following these principles, you can eat well and enjoy your food without compromising your health. You can also improve your blood sugar levels, lower your blood pressure, reduce your risk of complications, and enhance your well-being.

Benefits of Diabetic Renal Diet

1. **Lower blood pressure**: By limiting sodium, potassium, and fluids, you can reduce the pressure on your blood vessels and lower your risk of hypertension, stroke, and heart attack.

2. **Better blood sugar control**: By choosing healthy carbohydrates, limiting sugar, and eating consistent portions, you can prevent spikes and drops in your blood sugar levels and lower your risk of diabetes complications.

3. **Prevent kidney damage**: By limiting protein, phosphorus, and artificial phosphorus, you can reduce the workload on your kidneys and prevent further loss of kidney function.

4. **Prevent bone loss**: By limiting phosphorus and artificial phosphorus, you can prevent calcium from being pulled out of your bones and keep them strong and healthy.

5. **Prevent anemia**: By eating enough, but not too much protein, you can provide your body with enough iron and other nutrients to make red blood cells and prevent anemia.

6. **Prevent malnutrition:** By eating a balanced and varied diet that includes fruits, vegetables, whole grains, and healthy fats, you can ensure you get enough vitamins, minerals, antioxidants, and fiber to support your immune system, digestion & overall health.

7. **Improve quality of life**: By eating well and enjoying your food, you can feel more energetic, happier, and confident. You can also prevent or delay the need for dialysis or a kidney transplant.

Foods to Eat

Colorful Vegetables: Fill your plate with a variety of colorful vegetables such as leafy greens, broccoli, and bell peppers. These nutrient-rich options are low in calories and high in essential vitamins, minerals, and antioxidants.

Lean Proteins: Opt for lean protein sources like skinless poultry, fish, tofu, and legumes, these choices provide the necessary building blocks for muscle maintenance without overburdening the kidneys.

Whole Grains: Embrace whole grains like quinoa, brown rice, and whole wheat, which offer complex carbohydrates, fiber, and essential nutrients. They contribute to steady energy release and support digestive health.

Healthy Fats: Incorporate sources of healthy fats, such as avocados, nuts, and olive oil, these fats not only add richness to your meals but also provide essential fatty acids, promoting heart and overall health.

Low-Glycemic Fruits: Enjoy fruits with a low glycemic index, such as berries, cherries, and apples. These fruits release glucose slowly, preventing rapid spikes in blood sugar levels.

Dairy or Dairy Alternatives: Include moderate amounts of low-fat dairy or fortified dairy alternatives for calcium and vitamin D. Choose options that align with both diabetes and renal health guidelines.

Herbs and Spices: Enhance flavor without compromising health by using herbs and spices like basil, turmeric, and cinnamon. These additions not only contribute to taste but also offer potential anti-inflammatory and antioxidant benefits.

Foods to Avoid

High-Sugar Foods: Minimize the intake of sugary treats like candies, pastries, and sodas. Excessive sugar can lead to abrupt spikes in blood glucose levels, challenging diabetes management.

Processed Foods: Steer clear of heavily processed foods high in sodium, preservatives, and additives. These can contribute to elevated blood pressure, potentially impacting kidney function.

Red and Processed Meats: Limit the consumption of red and processed meats, as they may contain compounds that can strain the kidneys. Opt for leaner protein sources like poultry, fish, and plant-based alternatives instead.

High-Sodium Items: Reduce sodium intake by avoiding salty snacks, canned soups, and processed foods. Excessive sodium can elevate blood pressure, posing a risk to both cardiovascular and renal health.

High-Potassium Foods: For individuals with compromised kidney function, it's advisable to moderate intake of high-potassium foods like bananas, oranges, and tomatoes. These foods, while nutritious, can pose challenges for those with renal concerns.

Saturated and Trans Fats: Cut back on saturated and trans fats found in fried foods and commercially baked goods. These fats can contribute to inflammation and negatively impact heart health.

White Bread and Refined Grains: Opt for whole grains over refined grains like white bread, which can cause rapid spikes in blood sugar. Whole grains provide sustained energy & essential nutrients.

Comprehensive Shopping List for Diabetic Renal Diet

Produce Section:

- Leafy Greens (Spinach, Kale, Swiss Chard)
- Cruciferous Vegetables (Broccoli, Cauliflower)
- Bell Peppers
- Zucchini
- Cucumbers
- Tomatoes (moderate intake for potassium considerations)
- Avocados
- Berries (Strawberries, Blueberries, Raspberries)
- Cherries
- Apples (choose varieties lower in natural sugars)

Protein Sources:

- Skinless Poultry (Chicken, Turkey)
- Fish (Salmon, Cod, Tilapia)
- Tofu
- Lentils
- Chickpeas

Whole Grains and Legumes:

- Quinoa
- Brown Rice
- Whole Wheat Bread
- Oats
- Barley

Dairy or Dairy Alternatives:

- Low-Fat Yogurt
- Almond Milk (unsweetened, fortified)
- Cheese (moderate intake for phosphorus considerations)

Nuts and Seeds:

- Almonds
- Walnuts
- Chia Seeds
- Flaxseeds

Healthy Fats:

- Olive Oil
- Canola Oil

- Flaxseed Oil

Herbs and Spices:

- Basil
- Turmeric
- Cinnamon
- Garlic

Sweeteners (in moderation):

- Stevia
- Monk Fruit

CHAPTER 2

Breakfast Recipes for Diabetic Renal Diet

Yogurt Parfait with Granola & Berries

- **Preparation Time:** 5 minutes
- **Serves:** 1

Ingredients:

- 1 cup low-fat Greek yogurt
- 1/2 cup granola (low-sugar)
- 1/2 cup mixed berries (strawberries, blueberries, raspberries)
- 1 tablespoon honey or sugar substitute

Nutritional Information: Calories: 300 | Protein: 20g | Carbohydrates: 40g | Fat: 8g | Fiber: 6g

Instructions:

1. In a glass or bowl, layer half of the Greek yogurt.
2. Add a layer of half the granola on top of the yogurt.
3. Sprinkle half of the mixed berries over the granola.

4. Drizzle with half of the honey or sugar substitute.

5. Repeat the layers with the remaining ingredients.

6. Serve immediately and enjoy your nutritious Yogurt Parfait!

Serving Suggestions:

- Customize with additional fruits like sliced bananas or kiwi.

- Garnish with a sprinkle of chia seeds for added nutritional benefits.

- Pair with a side of whole grain toast for a well-balanced breakfast.

Egg White Omelet

- **Preparation Time:** 10 minutes
- **Serves:** 1

Ingredients:

- 3 egg whites
- 1/4 cup diced bell peppers
- 1/4 cup diced tomatoes
- 1/4 cup spinach, chopped
- 1 tablespoon feta cheese (optional)

- Salt and pepper to taste
- Cooking spray

Nutritional Information: Calories: 150 | Protein: 20g | Carbohydrates: 6g | Fat: 5g | Fiber: 2g

Instructions:

1. Heat a non-stick pan over medium heat, coat with cooking spray.
2. In a bowl, whisk the egg whites until frothy.
3. Pour the egg whites into the pan, spreading them evenly.
4. Sprinkle bell peppers, tomatoes, and spinach over one half of the omelet.
5. If desired, add feta cheese on top.
6. Once the edges set, carefully fold the omelet in half.
7. Season with salt and pepper, then cook until the cheese (if added) melts.
8. Serve hot and enjoy this protein-packed Egg White Omelet!

Serving Suggestions:

- Pair with a whole grain English muffin for a wholesome meal.
- Add a side of fresh fruit or a small salad for extra vitamins.
- Drizzle with hot sauce or salsa for a flavor kick without added sugars.

Crepes with Apples & Cinnamon

- **Preparation Time:** 20 minutes
- **Serves:** 2

Ingredients:

- 1 cup whole wheat flour
- 1 1/2 cups low-fat milk
- 2 eggs
- 1 tablespoon melted butter
- 2 apples, thinly sliced
- 1 teaspoon ground cinnamon
- 1 tablespoon honey or sugar substitute
- Cooking spray

Nutritional Information: Calories: 250 | Protein: 10g | Carbohydrates: 40g | Fat: 6g | Fiber: 6g

Instructions:

1. In a blender, combine flour, milk, eggs, and melted butter until smooth.
2. Heat a non-stick skillet over medium heat, coat with cooking spray.
3. Pour a small amount of batter into the pan, swirling to coat the bottom evenly, cook until the edges lift, flip, and cook the other side.
4. Repeat to make additional crepes.
5. In a separate pan, sauté apple slices with cinnamon until softened.
6. Spoon the apple mixture onto each crepe, fold, and drizzle with honey.
7. Serve warm and savor the delightful Crepes with Apples & Cinnamon!

Serving Suggestions:

- Dust with a sprinkle of powdered sugar for an extra touch.

- Pair with a dollop of Greek yogurt for added creaminess.
- Garnish with chopped nuts like almonds or pecans for texture.

English Muffin Breakfast Sandwich

- **Preparation Time:** 10 minutes
- **Serves:** 1

Ingredients:

1. 1 whole grain English muffin, split and toasted
2. 1 egg, fried or poached
3. 1 slice turkey or chicken bacon
4. 1 slice low-fat cheese (cheddar or Swiss)
5. 1 tomato slice
6. Fresh spinach leaves
7. Salt and pepper to taste

Nutritional Information: Calories: 300 | Protein: 18g | Carbohydrates: 30g | Fat: 12g | Fiber: 6g

Instructions:

1. Cook the bacon slice in a pan until crispy, then set aside.

2. In the same pan, fry or poach the egg to your preference.

3. Season the egg with salt and pepper during cooking.

4. Assemble the sandwich: Place the cooked egg on the bottom half of the toasted English muffin.

5. Add the bacon, cheese slice, tomato, and fresh spinach.

6. You can top with the other half of the English muffin.

7. Press gently to let the cheese melt slightly.

8. Serve warm and relish the wholesome English Muffin Breakfast Sandwich!

Serving Suggestions:

- Add a slice of avocado for extra creaminess and healthy fats.
- Serve with a side of mixed berries for a refreshing accompaniment.

- Enjoy with a cup of herbal tea or black coffee for a complete breakfast.

French Toast with Bananas, Walnuts & Maple Syrup

- **Preparation Time:** 15 minutes
- **Serves:** 2

Ingredients:

- 4 slices whole wheat bread
- 2 eggs
- 1/2 cup low-fat milk
- 1 teaspoon vanilla extract
- 1/2 teaspoon ground cinnamon
- Cooking spray
- 1 banana, sliced
- 2 tablespoons chopped walnuts
- 2 tablespoons sugar-free maple syrup

Nutritional Information: Calories: 280 | Protein: 10g | Carbohydrates: 35g | Fat: 12g | Fiber: 6g

Instructions:

1. Whisk eggs, milk, vanilla extract, and cinnamon together in a shallow dish.
2. Heat a non-stick skillet over medium heat, coat with cooking spray, dip each slice of bread into the egg mixture, ensuring both sides are coated.
3. Cook each slice until golden brown on both sides.
4. In a separate pan, lightly toast the chopped walnuts.
5. Serve the French toast topped with banana slices and toasted walnuts.
6. Drizzle with sugar-free maple syrup.
7. Enjoy this delightful French Toast with Bananas, Walnuts & Maple Syrup!

Serving Suggestions:

- Sprinkle with a dash of cinnamon for an extra layer of flavor.
- You can serve with a side of Greek yogurt for added protein.
- Garnish with a few fresh berries for a burst of freshness.

Spicy Tofu Scramblers

- **Preparation Time:** 15 minutes

- **Serves:** 2

Ingredients:

- 1 tablespoon olive oil
- 1/2 cup diced bell peppers
- 1/2 cup diced tomatoes
- 1/4 cup diced red onions
- 1 teaspoon turmeric powder
- 1/2 teaspoon cumin powder
- 1/4 teaspoon cayenne pepper (adjust to taste)
- 1 block firm tofu, crumbled
- Salt and pepper to taste
- Fresh cilantro for garnish

Nutritional Information: Calories: 180 | Protein: 14g | Carbohydrates: 8g | Fat: 10g | Fiber: 3g

Instructions:

1. Heat olive oil in a skillet over medium heat, sauté bell peppers, tomatoes, and red onions until softened.
2. Add turmeric, cumin, and cayenne pepper, stirring well.

3. Crumble the tofu into the skillet and mix until well combined, cook until tofu is heated through and slightly golden.
4. Season with salt and pepper to your preferred taste.
5. Garnish with fresh cilantro.
6. Serve hot, savoring the flavors of these Spicy Tofu Scramblers!

Serving Suggestions:

- Serve on whole grain toast for a complete breakfast.
- Top with sliced avocado for added creaminess.
- Pair with a side of salsa for an extra kick of flavor.

Breakfast Burritos

- **Preparation Time:** 20 minutes
- **Serves:** 2

Ingredients:

- 4 whole grain tortillas
- 4 large eggs, scrambled
- 1/2 cup black beans, drained and rinsed
- 1/2 cup diced tomatoes
- 1/4 cup diced red onions

- 1/4 cup shredded low-fat cheese
- 1 avocado, sliced
- Salsa for topping
- Fresh cilantro for garnish
- Cooking spray

Nutritional Information: Calories: 320 | Protein: 16g | Carbohydrates: 30g | Fat: 16g | Fiber: 8g

Instructions:

1. In a non-stick skillet, coat with cooking spray and scramble the eggs.
2. Warm the tortillas in the skillet or microwave.
3. Assemble each burrito: Place scrambled eggs in the center of a tortilla.
4. Add black beans, diced tomatoes, red onions, shredded cheese, and sliced avocado.
5. Top with salsa and fresh cilantro.
6. Fold the sides of the tortilla over the filling, then roll it up, repeat for the remaining burritos.
7. Serve warm and relish these wholesome Breakfast Burritos!

Serving Suggestions:

- You can add a dollop of Greek yogurt for extra creaminess.
- Serve with a side of fresh fruit salad for a burst of sweetness.
- Customize with your favorite hot sauce for an extra kick.

Lunch Recipes for Diabetic Renal Diet

Chicken Salad on Toast

- **Preparation Time:** 15 minutes
- **Serves:** 2

Ingredients:

1. 1 cup cooked chicken breast, shredded
2. 1/4 cup celery, finely chopped
3. 2 tablespoons red onion, finely diced
4. 2 tablespoons Greek yogurt
5. 1 tablespoon mayonnaise
6. 1 teaspoon Dijon mustard
7. Salt and pepper to taste
8. 4 slices whole grain bread, toasted

9. Fresh lettuce leaves for garnish

Nutritional Information: Calories: 250 | Protein: 20g | Carbohydrates: 20g | Fat: 10g | Fiber: 4g

Instructions:

1. In a bowl, combine shredded chicken, celery, and red onion.
2. In a separate bowl, mix Greek yogurt, mayonnaise, Dijon mustard, salt, and pepper.
3. Add the dressing to the chicken mixture, tossing until well coated.
4. Place a lettuce leaf on each slice of toasted whole grain bread.
5. Spoon the chicken salad onto the lettuce.
6. Top with additional lettuce leaves if desired.
7. Serve open-faced and enjoy your delicious Chicken Salad on Toast!

Serving Suggestions:

- Pair with a side of sliced tomatoes or cucumber for freshness.

- Add a sprinkle of chopped herbs like parsley or chives for extra flavor.
- Serve with a cup of vegetable soup for a wholesome lunch combination.

Lemony Hummus

- **Preparation Time:** 10 minutes
- **Serves:** 4

Ingredients:

- 15 oz (1 can) chickpeas, drained and rinsed
- 2 cloves garlic, minced
- 1/4 cup tahini
- 1/4 cup fresh lemon juice
- 2 tablespoons extra-virgin olive oil
- 1/2 teaspoon ground cumin
- Salt and pepper to taste
- Fresh parsley for garnish
- Whole grain pita or vegetable sticks for dipping

Nutritional Information: Calories: 150 | Protein: 5g | Carbohydrates: 15g | Fat: 8g | Fiber: 4g

Instructions:

1. In a food processor, combine chickpeas, minced garlic, tahini, lemon juice, olive oil, cumin, salt, and pepper.
2. Blend until smooth, scraping down the sides as needed, adjust seasoning to taste.
3. Transfer the hummus to a serving bowl.
4. Drizzle with a bit of olive oil and garnish with fresh parsley.
5. Serve with whole grain pita or vegetable sticks.

Serving Suggestions:

- Garnish with a sprinkle of paprika for a burst of color and flavor.
- Pair with cherry tomatoes and cucumber slices for a refreshing snack.
- Spread on whole grain crackers for a quick and satisfying lunch option.

Tuna Salad on Greens

- **Preparation Time:** 15 minutes
- **Serves:** 2

Ingredients:

- 5 oz (1 can) tuna in water, drained
- 2 cups mixed salad greens
- 1/2 cucumber, sliced
- 1/2 cup cherry tomatoes, halved
- 1/4 cup red onion, thinly sliced
- 2 tablespoons olive oil
- 1 tablespoon balsamic vinegar
- 1 teaspoon Dijon mustard
- Salt and pepper to taste
- Fresh basil for garnish

Nutritional Information: Calories: 280 | Protein: 20g | Carbohydrates: 10g | Fat: 18g | Fiber: 3g

Instructions:

1. In a bowl, combine drained tuna, salad greens, cucumber, cherry tomatoes, and red onion.
2. In a small jar, whisk together olive oil, balsamic vinegar, Dijon mustard, salt, and pepper to make the dressing.

3. Pour the dressing over the salad and toss gently to combine, then divide the salad onto two plates.

4. Top with tuna.

5. Garnish with fresh basil.

6. Serve immediately and relish the Tuna Salad on Greens!

Serving Suggestions:

- Add a sprinkle of pine nuts for extra crunch and healthy fats.

- Serve with a side of whole grain crackers for a complete meal.

- Drizzle with additional balsamic glaze for a flavor boost.

Buffalo Wings with Low Sodium Hot Sauce

- **Preparation Time:** 40 minutes
- **Serves:** 2

Ingredients:

- 1 lb chicken wings, split at joints, tips discarded

- 1/4 cup hot sauce (low sodium)
- 2 tablespoons unsalted butter, melted
- 1 tablespoon apple cider vinegar
- 1/2 teaspoon garlic powder
- 1/2 teaspoon onion powder
- 1/4 teaspoon cayenne pepper
- Celery sticks for serving
- Ranch or blue cheese dressing (optional)

Nutritional Information: Calories: 280 | Protein: 20g | Carbohydrates: 2g | Fat: 22g | Fiber: 0g

Instructions:

1. Preheat the oven to 400°F (200°C).
2. Place a wire rack on a baking sheet, pat dry chicken wings with paper towels and place them on the rack.
3. Bake wings for 35-40 minutes until golden and crispy.
4. In a bowl, mix hot sauce, melted butter, apple cider vinegar, garlic powder, onion powder, and cayenne pepper.
5. Toss baked wings in the sauce until evenly coated.
6. Transfer to a serving plate.

7. Serve with celery sticks and optional ranch or blue cheese dressing.

Serving Suggestions:

- Pair with a side of carrot sticks for additional crunch.
- Enjoy with a light, refreshing cucumber salad on the side.
- Serve as an appetizer or with a side of coleslaw for a complete meal.

Quinoa Tabbouleh Salad

- **Preparation Time:** 20 minutes
- **Serves:** 4

Ingredients:

- 1 cup quinoa, cooked and cooled
- 1 cucumber, diced
- 1 cup cherry tomatoes, halved
- 1/2 cup red onion, finely chopped
- 1/4 cup fresh parsley, chopped
- 1/4 cup fresh mint, chopped
- 1/4 cup olive oil

- 1/4 cup fresh lemon juice
- Salt and pepper to taste
- Crumbled feta cheese for garnish (optional)

Nutritional Information: Calories: 240 | Protein: 6g | Carbohydrates: 30g | Fat: 10g | Fiber: 5g

Instructions:

1. In a large bowl, combine quinoa, cucumber, cherry tomatoes, red onion, parsley, and mint.
2. In a small bowl, whisk together olive oil, lemon juice, salt, and pepper, pour the dressing over the quinoa mixture and toss to combine.
3. Garnish with crumbled feta cheese if desired.
4. Serve chilled and enjoy the refreshing Quinoa Tabbouleh Salad!

Serving Suggestions:

- Serve as a side dish with grilled chicken or fish.
- Spoon onto whole grain pita bread for a light lunch wrap.
- Top with grilled shrimp or tofu for an added protein boost.

Spicy Slaw Bowls with Shrimp & Edamame

- **Preparation Time:** 25 minutes
- **Serves:** 2

Ingredients:

- 1 cup shredded red cabbage
- 1 cup shredded green cabbage
- 1 cup cooked and peeled shrimp
- 1/2 cup shelled edamame, cooked
- 1/4 cup carrot, julienned
- 2 tablespoons low-sodium soy sauce
- 1 tablespoon sesame oil
- 1 tablespoon rice vinegar
- 1 teaspoon Sriracha sauce (adjust to taste)
- 1 tablespoon sesame seeds
- Fresh cilantro for garnish
- Brown rice or quinoa for serving

Nutritional Information: Calories: 320 | Protein: 25g | Carbohydrates: 20g | Fat: 15g | Fiber: 8g

Instructions:

1. In a large bowl, combine red cabbage, green cabbage, shrimp, edamame, and julienned carrot.
2. In a small bowl, whisk together soy sauce, sesame oil, rice vinegar, and Sriracha sauce.
3. Pour the dressing over the slaw mixture and toss until evenly coated.
4. Sprinkle sesame seeds and garnish with fresh cilantro.
5. You can serve over a bed of brown rice or quinoa.

Serving Suggestions:

- Top with sliced avocado for added creaminess.
- Garnish with a wedge of lime for a burst of citrus flavor.
- You can serve in lettuce wraps for a low-carb option.

Red Cabbage-Apple Cauliflower Gnocchi

- **Preparation Time:** 30 minutes
- **Serves:** 3

Ingredients:

- 1 package (16 oz) cauliflower gnocchi
- 2 cups red cabbage, thinly sliced
- 1 large apple, diced
- 1/4 cup red onion, finely chopped
- 2 tablespoons olive oil
- 1 tablespoon balsamic vinegar
- 1 tablespoon maple syrup
- Salt and pepper to taste
- Chopped pecans for garnish
- Fresh thyme for garnish

Nutritional Information: Calories: 280 | Protein: 5g | Carbohydrates: 45g | Fat: 9g | Fiber: 8g

Instructions:

1. Cook cauliflower gnocchi according to package instructions, then set aside.
2. In a large skillet, heat olive oil over medium heat, add red cabbage, apple, and red onion. Sauté until softened.
3. Stir in balsamic vinegar and maple syrup.

4. Add the cooked cauliflower gnocchi to the skillet, tossing to combine.

5. Season with salt and pepper to taste.

6. Garnish with chopped pecans and fresh thyme.

7. Serve warm and savor the unique flavors of Red Cabbage-Apple Cauliflower Gnocchi!

Serving Suggestions:

- Crumble feta or goat cheese on top for added creaminess.
- Serve with a side of mixed greens for extra freshness.
- Sprinkle with a dash of nutmeg for a hint of warmth.

Dinner Recipes for Diabetic Renal Diet

Cuban-Marinated Sirloin Kabobs with Grilled Asparagus

- **Preparation Time:** 30 minutes
- **Serves:** 4

Ingredients:

- 1 lb sirloin steak, cut into 1-inch cubes
- 1 bunch asparagus, trimmed
- 1/4 cup orange juice
- 2 tablespoons lime juice
- 2 tablespoons olive oil
- 2 cloves garlic, minced
- 1 teaspoon ground cumin
- 1 teaspoon dried oregano
- Salt and pepper to taste
- Wooden or metal skewers

Nutritional Information: Calories: 280 | Protein: 25g | Carbohydrates: 8g | Fat: 15g | Fiber: 4g

Instructions:

1. In a bowl, mix orange juice, lime juice, olive oil, minced garlic, ground cumin, dried oregano, salt, and pepper to create the marinade.
2. Place sirloin cubes in a zip-top bag, add half of the marinade, seal the bag, and marinate in the refrigerator for at least 20 minutes. preheat your grill or grill pan over medium-high heat.

3. Thread marinated sirloin cubes onto skewers, alternating with trimmed asparagus.

4. Grill kabobs for 8-10 minutes, turning occasionally until sirloin reaches desired doneness and asparagus is tender.

5. Baste with the reserved marinade during grilling, remove from the grill, let rest for a few minutes.

6. Serve hot and enjoy these flavorful Cuban-Marinated Sirloin Kabobs with Grilled Asparagus!

Serving Suggestions:

- You can serve over a bed of quinoa or brown rice for a complete meal.
- Decorate with fresh cilantro or parsley for a burst of freshness.
- Pair with a side of avocado salsa for added creaminess and flavor.

Stuffed Bell Peppers

- **Preparation Time:** 40 minutes
- **Serves:** 4

Ingredients:

1. 4 large bell peppers, halved & seeds completely removed
2. 1 lb lean ground turkey
3. 1 cup quinoa, cooked
4. 1 can (15 oz) black beans, drained and rinsed
5. 1 cup corn kernels (fresh or frozen)
6. 1 cup diced tomatoes
7. 1/2 cup diced red onion
8. 1 teaspoon ground cumin
9. 1 teaspoon chili powder
10. Salt and pepper to taste
11. 1 cup of shredded low-fat cheese (Mexican blend or cheddar)
12. Fresh cilantro for garnish

Nutritional Information: Calories: 350 | Protein: 25g | Carbohydrates: 40g | Fat: 10g | Fiber: 8g

Instructions:

- Preheat the oven to 375°F (190°C).
- In a skillet, cook ground turkey over medium heat until browned.

- In a large bowl, combine cooked turkey, quinoa, black beans, corn, diced tomatoes, red onion, cumin, chili powder, salt, and pepper.
- Spoon the mixture into halved bell peppers, pressing down gently.
- Top each stuffed pepper with shredded cheese.
- Place stuffed peppers in a baking dish, bake for 25-30 minutes or until peppers are tender.
- Garnish with fresh cilantro.
- Serve hot and savor these delicious Stuffed Bell Peppers!

Serving Suggestions:

- Serve with a side of salsa or guacamole for extra flavor.
- Pair with a side salad for a refreshing accompaniment.

Salmon and Rice Pilaf with Carrots and Peas

- **Preparation Time:** 25 minutes
- **Serves:** 2

Ingredients:

- 2 salmon fillets
- 1 cup brown rice, cooked
- 1/2 cup carrots, diced
- 1/2 cup peas
- 1/4 cup red onion, finely chopped
- 2 tablespoons olive oil
- 1 teaspoon garlic powder
- 1 teaspoon dried thyme
- Salt and pepper to taste
- Lemon wedges for garnish

Nutritional Information: Calories: 380 | Protein: 30g | Carbohydrates: 35g | Fat: 14g | Fiber: 6g

Instructions:

1. Preheat the oven to 375°F (190°C).
2. Place salmon fillets on a baking sheet lined with parchment paper, drizzle with olive oil and sprinkle with garlic powder, dried thyme, salt, and pepper.
3. Bake for 15-18 minutes or until salmon is cooked through.

4. In a skillet, sauté carrots and peas with red onion in olive oil until tender.

5. Stir in cooked brown rice and continue to cook for an additional 2-3 minutes.

6. Divide the rice pilaf between two plates, place a salmon fillet on top of each serving.

7. Garnish with lemon wedges.

8. Serve hot and enjoy this flavorful Salmon and Rice Pilaf with Carrots and Peas!

Serving Suggestions:

- Pair with a side of steamed broccoli for added nutrients.
- Drizzle with balsamic glaze for a touch of sweetness.
- Sprinkle with chopped fresh parsley for an extra burst of freshness.

Fish Tacos with Fresh Cabbage Slaw

- **Preparation Time:** 30 minutes
- **Serves:** 4

Ingredients:

For the Fish:

- 1 lb white fish fillets (tilapia or cod)
- 1 tablespoon olive oil
- 1 teaspoon chili powder
- 1/2 teaspoon cumin
- 1/2 teaspoon garlic powder
- Salt and pepper to taste

For the Cabbage Slaw:

- 2 cups shredded green cabbage
- 1 cup shredded purple cabbage
- 1/2 cup plain Greek yogurt
- 2 tablespoons lime juice
- 1 tablespoon honey
- 1/2 teaspoon cumin
- Salt and pepper to taste

For Assembly:

- 8 small whole wheat tortillas
- Fresh cilantro for garnish
- Lime wedges for serving

Nutritional Information: Calories: 320 | Protein: 25g | Carbohydrates: 30g | Fat: 10g | Fiber: 6g

Instructions:

1. Preheat the oven to 400°F (200°C).
2. Place fish fillets on a baking sheet lined with parchment paper.
3. Drizzle with olive oil and sprinkle with chili powder, cumin, garlic powder, salt, and pepper.
4. Bake for 13-15 minutes or until fish becomes flaky.
5. In a bowl, mix shredded green cabbage, purple cabbage, Greek yogurt, lime juice, honey, cumin, salt, and pepper to make the slaw.
6. Warm the tortillas in a dry skillet or microwave.
7. Assemble tacos with a layer of fish, a generous spoonful of cabbage slaw, and garnish with fresh cilantro.
8. Serve with lime wedges.
9. Enjoy these tasty Fish Tacos with Fresh Cabbage Slaw!

Serving Suggestions:

- Top with sliced avocado or guacamole for extra creaminess.
- Serve with a side of black beans for added protein and fiber.
- Drizzle with hot sauce for a spicy kick.

Thin Crust Pizza with Veggie Toppings & Tight Cheese

- **Preparation Time:** 40 minutes (including dough preparation)
- **Serves:** 3

Ingredients:

For the Pizza Dough:

- 2 1/4 cups whole wheat flour
- 1 teaspoon active dry yeast
- 1 teaspoon honey
- 1 cup warm water
- 1 tablespoon olive oil
- 1/2 teaspoon salt

For the Toppings:

- 1/2 cup tomato sauce (low sodium)
- 1 cup tight shredded mozzarella cheese
- 1/2 cup cherry tomatoes, sliced
- 1/2 cup bell peppers, thinly sliced
- 1/4 cup red onion, thinly sliced
- 1/4 cup black olives, sliced
- Fresh basil leaves for garnish

Nutritional Information: Calories: 300 | Protein: 15g | Carbohydrates: 40g | Fat: 10g | Fiber: 8g

Instructions:

For the Pizza Dough:

1. In a bowl, dissolve honey in warm water and sprinkle yeast over the top, tet it sit for 5-10 minutes until it becomes frothy.
2. In a large bowl, combine whole wheat flour and salt.
3. Pour the yeast mixture and olive oil into the flour. Mix until the dough comes together.

4. Knead the dough on a floured surface for 5-7 minutes until smooth.

5. Place the dough in a greased bowl, cover, and let it rise in a warm place for 30 minutes.

For the Pizza:

1. Preheat the oven to 475°F (245°C).

2. Roll out the pizza dough on a floured surface into a thin crust.

3. Transfer the crust to a pizza stone or baking sheet.

4. Spread a thin layer of tomato sauce over the crust.

5. Sprinkle shredded mozzarella evenly over the sauce.

6. Arrange sliced cherry tomatoes, bell peppers, red onion, and black olives on top.

7. Bake for 12-15 minutes or until the crust has turned to golden and the cheese is bubbly.

8. Garnish with fresh basil leaves.

9. Slice and enjoy this Thin Crust Pizza with Veggie Toppings & Tight Cheese!

Serving Suggestions:

- Drizzle with balsamic glaze for added sweetness.

- Top with arugula or spinach for extra greens.
- Serve with a side of mixed green salad for a complete meal.

Cobb Salad with Dijon Dressing

- **Preparation Time:** 20 minutes
- **Serves:** 2

Ingredients:

For the Salad:

- 2 cups mixed salad greens
- 1 cup cooked and diced chicken breast
- 1/2 cup cherry tomatoes, halved
- 1/2 cup cucumber, diced
- 1/4 cup crumbled feta cheese
- 2 hard-boiled eggs, sliced
- 1/4 cup crispy turkey bacon, crumbled
- 1/4 cup avocado, diced

For the Dijon Dressing:

- 2 tablespoons olive oil
- 1 tablespoon Dijon mustard

- 1 tablespoon red wine vinegar
- 1 teaspoon honey
- Salt and pepper to taste

Nutritional Information: Calories: 380 | Protein: 25g | Carbohydrates: 15g | Fat: 25g | Fiber: 6g

Instructions:

1. In a large bowl, arrange mixed salad greens as the base.
2. Top with diced chicken breast, cherry tomatoes, cucumber, crumbled feta cheese, sliced hard-boiled eggs, crispy turkey bacon, and diced avocado.
3. In a small jar, whisk together olive oil, Dijon mustard, red wine vinegar, honey, salt, and pepper to make the dressing.
4. Drizzle the dressing over the salad.
5. Toss gently to coat all the ingredients.
6. Serve immediately and relish the flavors of this Cobb Salad with Dijon Dressing!

Serving Suggestions:

- Add a handful of nuts (walnuts or pecans) for extra crunch.
- Pair with a side of whole grain bread or a breadstick.
- Customize with your favorite vegetables like bell peppers or red onion.

Grilled Shrimp Skewers

- **Preparation Time:** 20 minutes
- **Serves:** 4

Ingredients:

For the Shrimp Marinade:

- 1 lb large shrimp, peeled and deveined
- 2 tablespoons olive oil
- 2 tablespoons fresh lemon juice
- 2 cloves garlic, minced
- 1 teaspoon dried oregano
- Salt and pepper to taste

For the Skewers:

- Wooden or metal skewers

- Cherry tomatoes
- Red bell pepper, cut into chunks
- Red onion, cut into chunks
- Zucchini, sliced

Nutritional Information: Calories: 180 | Protein: 20g | Carbohydrates: 5g | Fat: 8g | Fiber: 2g

Instructions:

For the Shrimp Marinade:

1. In a bowl, mix olive oil, fresh lemon juice, minced garlic, dried oregano, salt, and pepper to create the marinade.
2. Add peeled and deveined shrimp to the marinade, ensuring they are well coated.
3. Cover and refrigerate for at least 30 minutes, allowing the flavors to meld.

For the Skewers:

1. Preheat the grill or grill pan over medium-high heat, thread marinated shrimp, cherry tomatoes, red bell pepper chunks, red onion chunks, and zucchini slices onto skewers.

2. Grill skewers for 5-7 minutes, turning occasionally, until shrimp are opaque and vegetables are tender, remove from the grill and serve immediately.

Serving Suggestions:

- Serve over a bed of quinoa or brown rice for a wholesome meal.
- Drizzle with a squeeze of fresh lemon juice before serving.
- Pair with a side of Greek salad for a Mediterranean twist.

Desserts and Snacks for Diabetic Renal Diet

Strawberry Fruit Salad

- **Preparation Time:** 15 minutes
- **Serves:** 4

Ingredients:

- 2 cups fresh strawberries, hulled and halved
- 1 cup fresh blueberries
- 1 cup fresh pineapple chunks

- 1 cup green grapes, halved
- 1 tablespoon honey
- 1 tablespoon fresh mint, finely chopped
- 1 tablespoon lime juice

Nutritional Information: Calories: 80 | Protein: 1g | Carbohydrates: 20g | Fat: 0.5g | Fiber: 4g

Instructions:

1. In a large bowl, combine fresh strawberries, blueberries, pineapple chunks, and halved green grapes.
2. In a small bowl, whisk together honey and lime juice to create the dressing.
3. Pour the dressing over the fruit and toss gently to coat.
4. Sprinkle finely chopped fresh mint over the salad and toss again.
5. Chill in the refrigerator for at least 10 minutes before serving to enhance flavors.
6. Serve the refreshing Strawberry Fruit Salad in individual bowls or as a side dish.

Serving Suggestions:

- You can top with a dollop of Greek yogurt for added creaminess.
- Garnish with a sprinkle of toasted almonds or coconut flakes.

Unsalted Crackers with Almond Butter

- **Preparation Time:** 5 minutes
- **Serves:** 2

Ingredients:

- 8 unsalted whole grain crackers
- 4 tablespoons almond butter

Nutritional Information: Calories: 260 | Protein: 8g | Carbohydrates: 20g | Fat: 16g | Fiber: 4g

Instructions:

1. Place unsalted whole grain crackers on a serving plate.
2. Spoon almond butter into a small bowl for easy spreading.
3. Spread a generous layer of almond butter onto each cracker.

4. Arrange the crackers on a plate for serving.

5. Serve the Unsalted Crackers with Almond Butter as a quick and satisfying snack.

Serving Suggestions:

- Top with banana slices for added sweetness and potassium.

- Enjoy with a side of Greek yogurt for a protein boost.

Vanilla Pudding with Coconut Milk

- **Preparation Time:** 15 minutes
- **Serves:** 4

Ingredients:

- 1 can (14 oz) coconut milk
- 1/4 cup cornstarch
- 1/3 cup granulated sugar
- 1/4 teaspoon salt
- 2 teaspoons vanilla extract
- Shredded coconut for garnish (optional)

Nutritional Information: Calories: 200 | Protein: 1g | Carbohydrates: 20g | Fat: 14g | Fiber: 1g

Instructions:

- In a small bowl, mix cornstarch with a couple of tablespoons of coconut milk to create a smooth paste.
- In a saucepan, combine the remaining coconut milk, granulated sugar, and salt. Heat over medium heat until it begins to simmer.
- Slowly whisk in the cornstarch paste, stirring constantly to avoid lumps.
- Continue to cook and stir until the mixture thickens, remove from heat and stir in vanilla extract.
- Pour the pudding into serving bowls and let it cool to room temperature.
- Refrigerate for at least 2 hours until the pudding is set.
- Garnish with shredded coconut before serving, if desired.
- Serve and savor the delightful Vanilla Pudding with Coconut Milk!

Serving Suggestions:

- Top with a dollop of dairy-free whipped cream for added richness.
- Sprinkle with ground cinnamon or nutmeg for a warm flavor.
- Pair with fresh berries or sliced banana for a fruity twist.

Baked Apple Crisp

- **Preparation Time:** 40 minutes
- **Serves:** 6

Ingredients:

For the Apple Filling:

- 6 medium-sized apples, peeled, cored, and sliced
- 2 tablespoons lemon juice
- 1/4 cup granulated sugar
- 1 teaspoon ground cinnamon
- 1/4 teaspoon nutmeg

For the Crisp Topping:

- 1 cup old-fashioned oats

- 1/2 cup whole wheat flour
- 1/4 cup chopped nuts (almonds or walnuts)
- 1/4 cup melted coconut oil
- 1/4 cup pure maple syrup
- 1/2 teaspoon vanilla extract
- Pinch of salt

Nutritional Information: Calories: 220 | Protein: 3g | Carbohydrates: 38g | Fat: 8g | Fiber: 6g

Instructions:

For the Apple Filling:

- Preheat the oven to 350°F (175°C).
- In a large bowl, toss sliced apples with lemon juice, granulated sugar, ground cinnamon, and nutmeg.
- Transfer the apple mixture to a baking dish.

For the Crisp Topping:

1. In a separate bowl, combine oats, whole wheat flour, chopped nuts, melted coconut oil, maple syrup, vanilla extract, and a pinch of salt. Mix until crumbly.

2. Sprinkle the crisp topping evenly over the apple mixture.
3. Bake for 25-30 minutes or until the topping is golden brown, and the apples are tender.
4. Allow the Baked Apple Crisp to cool slightly before serving.

Serving Suggestions:

- Serve warm with a scoop of vanilla frozen yogurt or a dollop of whipped cream.
- Garnish with additional chopped nuts for added crunch.

Almond Vegan Ice Cream

- **Preparation Time:** 10 minutes
- **Serves:** 4

Ingredients:

- 2 cans (28 oz) full-fat coconut milk
- 1 cup almond milk
- 1 cup granulated sugar
- Pinch of salt
- Sliced almonds for garnish (optional)

Nutritional Information: Calories: 300 | Protein: 2g | Carbohydrates: 30g | Fat: 20g | Fiber: 1g

Instructions:

1. In a blender, combine coconut milk, almond milk, granulated sugar, and a pinch of salt.
2. Blend until the mixture is smooth, pour the mixture into an ice cream maker and churn according to the manufacturer's instructions.
3. Transfer the churned ice cream to a lidded container, sprinkle sliced almonds if desired, and freeze for at least 4 hours.
4. Scoop and enjoy this creamy Almond Vegan Ice Cream guilt-free!

Serving Suggestions:

- Serve in a gluten-free cone for a crunchy texture.
- Drizzle with dairy-free chocolate sauce for added indulgence.
- Top with fresh berries for a fruity twist.

Beverages/Drinks for Diabetic Renal Diet

Lemon Lavender Herbal Tea

- **Preparation Time:** 10 minutes
- **Serves:** 2

Ingredients:

- 2 cups water
- 2 teaspoons dried lavender buds
- 2 teaspoons dried chamomile flowers
- 2 teaspoons honey (optional)
- 1 lemon, sliced
- Fresh lavender sprigs for garnish (optional)

Nutritional Information: Calories: 10 | Protein: 0g | Carbohydrates: 3g | Fat: 0g | Fiber: 1g

Instructions:

1. In a pot, bring 2 cups of water to a gentle boil.

2. Remove the water from heat and add dried lavender buds and chamomile flowers to the hot water.

3. Let the herbs steep for 5-7 minutes, allowing the flavors to infuse.

4. Strain the tea into serving cups, discarding the herbs.

5. Add honey to the tea if desired, stirring until it dissolves.

6. Squeeze lemon slices into the tea and drop them into the cups.

7. Garnish with fresh lavender sprigs for a fragrant touch.

8. Serve the soothing Lemon Lavender Herbal Tea immediately.

Serving Suggestions:

- Pair with a light and kidney-friendly snack like unsalted almonds.

- Enjoy as an afternoon pick-me-up or wind-down in the evening.

- Serve over ice for a refreshing iced version during warmer days.

Peach Iced Tea

- **Preparation Time:** 15 minutes
- **Serves:** 4

Ingredients:

- 4 cups water
- 4 black tea bags
- 2 ripe peaches, sliced
- 2 tablespoons honey (optional)
- Fresh mint leaves for garnish
- Ice cubes

Nutritional Information: Calories: 15 | Protein: 0g | Carbohydrates: 4g | Fat: 0g | Fiber: 0g

Instructions:

1. In a saucepan, bring 4 cups of water to a boil, remove the saucepan from heat, add black tea bags
2. Steep for 5-7 minutes, then discard the tea bags and let the tea cool to room temperature.
3. In a blender, puree the sliced peaches until smooth.

4. Combine the peach puree with the cooled black tea.

5. Add honey if a sweeter taste is desired, stirring until well combined.

6. Chill the Peach Iced Tea in the refrigerator for at least 2 hours, serve over ice, garnished with fresh mint leaves.

Serving Suggestions:

- Garnish with peach slices for an extra visual appeal.
- Serve with a wedge of lemon for a citrusy twist.
- Enjoy alongside a kidney-friendly sandwich for a light lunch.

Spiced Chai

- **Preparation Time:** 15 minutes
- **Serves:** 2

Ingredients:

- 2 cups water
- 2 black tea bags
- 1 cup unsweetened almond milk
- 1 cinnamon stick
- 4 whole cloves

- 4 cardamom pods, lightly crushed
- 1-inch fresh ginger, sliced
- 1-2 tablespoons honey (optional)

Nutritional Information: Calories: 20 | Protein: 1g | Carbohydrates: 3g | Fat: 1g | Fiber: 1g

Instructions:

1. In a saucepan, bring 2 cups of water to a boil, remove the saucepan from heat, add black tea bags, and steep for 3-5 minutes.
2. In the same saucepan, add almond milk, cinnamon stick, cloves, crushed cardamom pods, and sliced ginger.
3. Bring the mixture to a gentle simmer over medium heat, allowing the spices to infuse.
4. Remove from heat and let the chai steep for an additional 5 minutes.
5. Strain the spiced chai into serving cups.
6. Add honey if desired, stirring until dissolved.
7. Serve the comforting Spiced Chai hot.

Serving Suggestions:

- Dust with a pinch of ground cinnamon for added aroma.
- Enjoy with a kidney-friendly cookie or biscuit on the side.
- Serve in a traditional chai cup for an authentic experience.

Ginger Ale

- **Preparation Time:** 10 minutes
- **Serves:** 2

Ingredients:

- 2 cups sparkling water
- 2 tablespoons fresh ginger, grated
- 1-2 tablespoons honey (adjust to taste)
- 1 lemon, juiced
- Ice cubes
- Fresh mint leaves for garnish

Nutritional Information: Calories: 30 | Protein: 0g | Carbohydrates: 8g | Fat: 0g | Fiber: 0g

Instructions:

- In a small bowl, combine grated fresh ginger and honey. Mix well to create a ginger-infused sweetener.
- In serving glasses, add ice cubes.
- Pour sparkling water over the ice in each glass.
- Squeeze fresh lemon juice into the glasses, adjusting to taste.
- Add the prepared ginger-infused sweetener to each glass, stirring until well combined.
- Decorate with fresh mint leaves for a burst of flavor.
- Serve the refreshing Ginger Ale immediately.

Serving Suggestions:

- Add a slice of cucumber for a cool and crisp variation.
- Enjoy with a kidney-friendly salad for a light meal.

- Customize sweetness by adjusting the honey to suit personal preferences.

Tropical Fruit Punch

- **Preparation Time:** 15 minutes (plus chilling time)
- **Serves:** 4

Ingredients:

- 2 cups pineapple juice, unsweetened
- 1 cup mango juice, unsweetened
- 1 cup passion fruit juice, unsweetened
- 1 lime, juiced
- 1-2 tablespoons agave syrup (adjust to taste)
- Pineapple slices and mint leaves for garnish
- Ice cubes

Nutritional Information: Calories: 80 | Protein: 1g | Carbohydrates: 20g | Fat: 0.5g | Fiber: 1g

Instructions:

1. In a large pitcher, combine pineapple juice, mango juice, passion fruit juice, and fresh lime juice.

2. Stir in agave syrup, adjusting sweetness to your liking.

3. Chill the Tropical Fruit Punch in the refrigerator for at least 2 hours.

4. Before serving, add ice cubes to individual glasses, pour the fruit punch over the ice in each glass.

5. Garnish with pineapple slices and mint leaves for a tropical touch.

6. Serve the vibrant Tropical Fruit Punch immediately.

Serving Suggestions:

- You can add a splash of sparkling water for a fizzy version.

- Pair with a kidney-friendly fruit salad for a refreshing snack.

- Serve in decorative glasses for a festive presentation.

CHAPTER 3

30 Days Meal Plan for Diabetic Renal Diet

Please note that the provided meal plan is a sample and should not be interpreted as a recommendation to consume all the listed recipes in a single day.

This meal plan aims to offer inspiration and guidance for healthy meal preparation. Feel free to customize this plan to suit your preferences and dietary requirements.

Day 1:

- **Breakfast:** Yogurt Parfait with Granola & Berries
- **Lunch:** Chicken Salad on Toast
- **Dinner:** Cuban-Marinated Sirloin Kabobs with Grilled Asparagus
- **Beverage:** Lemon Lavender Herbal Tea

Day 2:

- **Breakfast:** Egg White Omelet
- **Lunch:** Lemony Hummus
- **Dinner:** Stuffed Bell Peppers

- **Beverage:** Peach Iced Tea

Day 3:

- **Breakfast:** Crepes with Apples & Cinnamon
- **Lunch:** Tuna Salad on Greens
- **Dinner:** Salmon and Rice Pilaf with Carrots and Peas
- **Beverage:** Spiced Chai

Day 4:

- **Breakfast:** English Muffin Breakfast Sandwich
- **Lunch:** Buffalo Wings with Low Sodium Hot Sauce
- **Dinner:** Fish Tacos with Fresh Cabbage Slaw
- **Beverage:** Ginger Ale

Day 5:

- **Breakfast:** French Toast with Bananas, Walnuts & Maple Syrup
- **Lunch:** Quinoa Tabbouleh Salad
- **Dinner:** Thin Crust Pizza with Veggie Toppings & Tight Cheese
- **Beverage:** Tropical Fruit Punch

Day 6:

- **Breakfast:** Spicy Tofu Scramblers
- **Lunch:** Spicy Slaw Bowls with Shrimp and Edamame
- **Dinner:** Cobb Salad with Dijon Dressing
- **Beverage:** Vanilla Pudding with Coconut Milk

Day 7:

- **Breakfast:** Breakfast Burritos
- **Lunch:** Red Cabbage-Apple Cauliflower Gnocchi
- **Dinner:** Grilled Shrimp Skewers
- **Beverage:** Chia Seed Pudding with Mixed Berries

Day 8:

- **Breakfast:** Yogurt Parfait with Granola & Berries
- **Lunch:** Chicken Salad on Toast
- **Dinner:** Cuban-Marinated Sirloin Kabobs with Grilled Asparagus
- **Beverage:** Lemon Lavender Herbal Tea

Day 9:

- **Breakfast:** Egg White Omelet

- **Lunch:** Lemony Hummus
- **Dinner:** Stuffed Bell Peppers
- **Beverage:** Peach Iced Tea

Day 10:

- **Breakfast:** Crepes with Apples & Cinnamon
- **Lunch:** Tuna Salad on Greens
- **Dinner:** Salmon and Rice Pilaf with Carrots and Peas
- **Beverage:** Spiced Chai

Day 11:

- **Breakfast:** English Muffin Breakfast Sandwich
- **Lunch:** Buffalo Wings with Low Sodium Hot Sauce
- **Dinner:** Fish Tacos with Fresh Cabbage Slaw
- **Beverage:** Ginger Ale

Day 12:

- **Breakfast:** French Toast with Bananas, Walnuts & Maple Syrup
- **Lunch:** Quinoa Tabbouleh Salad

- **Dinner:** Thin Crust Pizza with Veggie Toppings & Tight Cheese
- **Beverage:** Tropical Fruit Punch

Day 13:

- **Breakfast:** Spicy Tofu Scramblers
- **Lunch:** Spicy Slaw Bowls with Shrimp and Edamame
- **Dinner:** Cobb Salad with Dijon Dressing
- **Beverage:** Vanilla Pudding with Coconut Milk

Day 14:

- **Breakfast:** Breakfast Burritos
- **Lunch:** Red Cabbage-Apple Cauliflower Gnocchi
- **Dinner:** Grilled Shrimp Skewers
- **Beverage:** Chia Seed Pudding with Mixed Berries

Day 15:

- **Breakfast:** Crepes with Apples & Cinnamon
- **Lunch:** Tuna Salad on Greens
- **Dinner:** Salmon and Rice Pilaf with Carrots and Peas
- **Beverage:** Spiced Chai

Day 16:

- **Breakfast:** Yogurt Parfait with Granola & Berries
- **Lunch:** Chicken Salad on Toast
- **Dinner:** Cuban-Marinated Sirloin Kabobs with Grilled Asparagus
- **Beverage:** Lemon Lavender Herbal Tea

Day 17:

- **Breakfast:** Egg White Omelet
- **Lunch:** Lemony Hummus
- **Dinner:** Stuffed Bell Peppers
- **Beverage:** Peach Iced Tea

Day 18:

- **Breakfast:** Crepes with Apples & Cinnamon
- **Lunch:** Tuna Salad on Greens
- **Dinner:** Salmon and Rice Pilaf with Carrots and Peas
- **Beverage:** Spiced Chai

Day 19:

- **Breakfast:** English Muffin Breakfast Sandwich
- **Lunch:** Buffalo Wings with Low Sodium Hot Sauce
- **Dinner:** Fish Tacos with Fresh Cabbage Slaw
- **Beverage:** Ginger Ale

Day 20:

- **Breakfast:** French Toast with Bananas, Walnuts & Maple Syrup
- **Lunch:** Quinoa Tabbouleh Salad
- **Dinner:** Thin Crust Pizza with Veggie Toppings & Tight Cheese
- **Beverage:** Tropical Fruit Punch

Day 21:

- **Breakfast:** Spicy Tofu Scramblers
- **Lunch:** Spicy Slaw Bowls with Shrimp and Edamame
- **Dinner:** Cobb Salad with Dijon Dressing
- **Beverage:** Vanilla Pudding with Coconut Milk

Day 22:

- **Breakfast:** Breakfast Burritos

- **Lunch:** Red Cabbage-Apple Cauliflower Gnocchi
- **Dinner:** Grilled Shrimp Skewers
- **Beverage:** Chia Seed Pudding with Mixed Berries

Day 23:

- **Breakfast:** Yogurt Parfait with Granola & Berries
- **Lunch:** Chicken Salad on Toast
- **Dinner:** Cuban-Marinated Sirloin Kabobs with Grilled Asparagus
- **Beverage:** Lemon Lavender Herbal Tea

Day 24:

- **Breakfast:** Egg White Omelet
- **Lunch:** Lemony Hummus
- **Dinner:** Stuffed Bell Peppers
- **Beverage:** Peach Iced Tea

Day 25:

- **Breakfast:** Crepes with Apples & Cinnamon
- **Lunch:** Tuna Salad on Greens
- **Dinner:** Salmon and Rice Pilaf with Carrots and Peas
- **Beverage:** Spiced Chai

Day 26:

- **Breakfast:** English Muffin Breakfast Sandwich
- **Lunch:** Buffalo Wings with Low Sodium Hot Sauce
- **Dinner:** Fish Tacos with Fresh Cabbage Slaw
- **Beverage:** Ginger Ale

Day 27:

- **Breakfast:** French Toast with Bananas, Walnuts & Maple Syrup
- **Lunch:** Quinoa Tabbouleh Salad
- **Dinner:** Thin Crust Pizza with Veggie Toppings & Tight Cheese
- **Beverage:** Tropical Fruit Punch

Day 28:

- **Breakfast:** Spicy Tofu Scramblers
- **Lunch:** Spicy Slaw Bowls with Shrimp and Edamame
- **Dinner:** Cobb Salad with Dijon Dressing
- **Beverage:** Vanilla Pudding with Coconut Milk

Day 29:

- **Breakfast:** Breakfast Burritos
- **Lunch:** Red Cabbage-Apple Cauliflower Gnocchi
- **Dinner:** Grilled Shrimp Skewers
- **Beverage:** Chia Seed Pudding with Mixed Berries

Day 30:

- **Breakfast:** Yogurt Parfait with Granola & Berries
- **Lunch:** Chicken Salad on Toast
- **Dinner:** Cuban-Marinated Sirloin Kabobs with Grilled Asparagus
- **Beverage:** Lemon Lavender Herbal Tea

CHAPTER 4

Conclusion

In concluding this Diabetic Renal Diet Cookbook, we embark on a flavorful journey that transcends the boundaries of health and culinary delight.

Through the carefully crafted recipes and comprehensive meal plans, we have navigated the intricacies of managing diabetes and renal health with a focus on nourishment and indulgence.

This cookbook is more than a compilation of recipes; it is a testament to the power of conscious eating.

By adhering to the principles of the Diabetic Renal Diet, we have discovered a harmonious balance between flavors, nutrition, and well-being.

Each dish is not just a culinary creation; it is a step towards nurturing the body, respecting its needs, and savoring the joy that comes from wholesome, kidney-friendly meals. The benefits of this cookbook extend beyond the kitchen.

We have explored the profound impact of mindful food choices on overall health, emphasizing the positive outcomes of adopting a Diabetic Renal Diet.

From controlling blood sugar levels to supporting kidney function, every recipe plays a crucial role in facing the dual challenge of diabetes and renal concerns.

The journey doesn't end with the last page; it merely marks the beginning of a sustainable and enriching lifestyle.

Armed with a comprehensive shopping list, diverse meal plans, and an arsenal of breakfasts, lunches, dinners, desserts, and beverages, you can embrace variety and excitement in their daily culinary experiences.

The 30-day meal plan serves as a guide, ensuring that every day brings a new opportunity to delight the taste buds and nurture the body.

As we close the pages of this cookbook, let it be a reminder that healthful eating need not sacrifice taste.

It is an invitation to explore, experiment, and relish the delightful union of flavors that align with the principles of the Diabetic Renal Diet.

May this cookbook be a constant companion in your culinary endeavors, fostering a joyful relationship with food and, most importantly, cultivating a path to lasting wellness.

www.ingramcontent.com/pod-product-compliance
Lightning Source LLC
Chambersburg PA
CBHW071059290526
45795CB00004B/1572